0000774

The Library
Education & Training Centre
Tunbridge Wells Hospital
Tonbridge Road
Pembury
Kent TN2 4QJ

# TEAM BUILDING IN PRIMARY HEALTH CARE:
## AN EVALUATION

The Library
Education & Training Centre
Tunbridge Wells Hospital
Tonbridge Road
Pembury
Kent TN2 4QJ

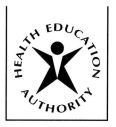

# TEAM BUILDING IN PRIMARY HEALTH CARE: AN EVALUATION

## Michael A West

Professor of Work and Organisational Psychology
Institute of Work Psychology
University of Sheffield

and

## Tracey Pillinger

Research Scientist
Institute of Work Psychology
University of Sheffield

SCHOOL OF NURSING

LIBRARY

PEMBURY HOSPITAL

A report prepared for the Health Education Authority

PN
12307

*Acknowledgements*

We acknowledge with thanks the assistance of those within many NHS and university sector organisations who responded to our requests for information in the preparation of this report. In particular, the help of local organising team members was invaluable. Our thanks also to Sue Potter and Pamela Baxter of the HEA, whose support and gentle steers helped us to stay on course.

W 89.3
W 93

PRIMARY
H C TEAMS
TEAM BUILDING

Published by the Health Education Authority

ISBN 0 7521 0664 3

© Health Education Authority 1996
First published 1996

Health Education Authority
Hamilton House
Mabledon Place
London WC1H 9TX

Typeset by DP Photosetting, Aylesbury, Bucks
Printed in England

# Contents

Acknowledgements                                                                iv

Summary                                                                          1

The aim of this review                                                           3

How the review was carried out                                                   4

What is team building?                                                           5

Types of team intervention                                                       7
1. Team member selection                                                         7
2. Team building                                                                 8
3. Team training                                                                 9
4. Leadership training                                                          10
5. Work re-design                                                               10
6. Organisational context interventions                                        11

The HEA Multidisciplinary Team Workshop Programme                              13

LOT representatives' descriptions of their team-building exercises             15
Models, methods and content                                                     15
Attendance at workshops                                                         16
The venue                                                                       17
Effectiveness of team-building workshops                                        17

Evaluation of workshops by LOTs                                                21

Examples of good practice                                                       23
1. Primary Health Care Team Development Programme –
   United Health Commission                                                     23
2. Team Care Valleys Initiative                                                 24
3. Multidisciplinary Audit                                                      25
4. Team Building in Primary Care – Cheshire Community Health                    26
5. The Micropurchasing Project – Northern and Yorkshire Region                 26
6. The King's Fund Organisation Audit (KFOA)                                    28
7. Primary Care Team Development – Dorset Health                                29

Conclusions and recommendations                                                31
1. Clarity of team objectives                                                   32
2. Participation                                                                32
3. Task orientation                                                             33
4. Support for innovation                                                       33

Further reading                                                                 35

*Contents*

**References**     37

**Appendices**
A   How this review was conducted     39
B   The LOT Teamworking Questionnaire     41

# Summary

- The purpose of this review is to describe and evaluate team-building methods which can be used in primary health care settings. In particular, the work of local organising teams (LOTs) from the HEA Multidisciplinary Team Workshop (MDTW) Programme is examined.

- Among the approaches used for making teams effective are team member selection, process interventions in building team relationships, team training, leadership development, teamwork re-design and changing the organisational context. Their use depends upon the particular needs of teams, the context in which they operate, and their stage of development. Appropriate diagnosis of team needs is therefore important.

- The MDTW Programme's team-building workshops have had a major influence upon the development of teamwork in primary health care.

- These workshops emphasise most areas such as building relationships, cohesion, collaboration and mutual role understanding. Least emphasised are disease prevention, relationships with patients, health promotion and health needs assessment. This suggests a predominant focus on relationship rather than task-related issues.

- Most LOT workshops involve only a sub-sample of team members, with consequent difficulties in exporting changed attitudes and innovative action plans to the rest of the primary health care team.

- Other areas LOT representatives identified as requiring particular improvement were better workshop planning and team diagnosis, better uptake of workshops by teams, developing advanced workshops using alternative models of team building, more resources, training and recognition for LOTs, measurable objectives for teams and post-workshop follow-up.

- In general, LOT workshops did not address the areas of future key demands on primary health care teams that LOT members themselves identified.

- Considerable and valuable evaluation of the workshops is being undertaken, though this is largely impressionistic and lacks empirical validation. Those empirical evaluations which have been undertaken suggest that team building has an impact upon both attitudes and team processes. However, impacts upon effectiveness of primary health care have not been identified.

- A number of examples of good practice exist which can inform LOTs of the types of alternative models of team development available.

- There is a need now for more advanced approaches to team building in this context which focus on developing clear, agreed long-term strategies for addressing the health needs of local populations, practice planning, decision-making and reviewing policies, practices and procedures.

- In particular, there is no clear model of leadership in primary health care teams and many fail to hold even regular team meetings to set objectives and review functioning. Moreover, training in teamwork and organisational functioning is needed by most primary health care team members.

● Overall, there is a need to develop ways of working which encourage continual team review and modification of objectives, strategies and processes in order that team members can effectively meet the changing health care needs of their local populations.

# The aim of this review

The purpose of this review is to describe and evaluate team-building methods currently employed in health care and elsewhere. In particular, team-building methods employed by local organising teams (LOTs) are examined. The report also identifies key issues to be addressed in the developing strategy of promoting team building in primary health care. The report provides LOTs and potential clients of the Health Education Authority, such as purchasers and commissioners, with information which will support the continuing development of the Multidisciplinary Team Workshop (MDTW) Programme as a method of team development in primary health care.

The HEA MDTW Programme was initiated in 1987 and has been supported by the HEA National Unit for Health Promotion in Primary Care in Oxford since 1989. The programme exists to support multidisciplinary team building in primary health care teams by the provision of team-building workshops. These are provided locally by LOTs. LOTs themselves are multidisciplinary teams whose membership reflects a multi-agency commitment and approach to developing primary health care in their locality. Their membership can consist of a range of professionals, including those from general practices, health authorities (FHSAs/DHAs), higher education, local authority and voluntary organisations. There have been around 70 LOTs operating in England and over 350 primary health care team-building workshops have been run which translates to direct training for over 1700 primary health care professionals, with many more members of primary health care teams receiving feedback and information from colleagues who attended the workshops.

The nature of HEA support has been reviewed at intervals since 1989, in consultation with LOT members and other key professionals working in primary care. The latest consultation exercise took place at a strategy and development workshop in June 1994. The report of the exercise, with the results and key findings, describes the areas of need highlighted by LOTs, including the need for further research and information on team building (HEA, 1995). In particular, LOTs identified the need for research on the advantages and disadvantages of the various models of team building. LOTs felt that further evaluation such as this would help them to influence managers to support team-building activities, to secure funds, influence purchasers and recruit primary health care teams.

The overall aim of this review is therefore to provide a clear and accessible description of models of team building available to LOTs and purchasers along with an analysis of the relative strengths of these approaches.

# How the review was carried out

There were four main components to the methodology of this review:

- a review of the literature on team-building methods used in organisational psychology, management science and organisational behaviour
- a review of research literature on team building in health care settings, particularly focused on primary health care
- a survey of LOTs and interview with LOT representatives to determine the models of team building employed and LOT evaluations of the effectiveness of those interventions
- a survey of team-building models employed in other health care settings via consultancies, NHS contacts and university departments of general practice.

Further details of the methodology of the reviews are given in Appendix A.

This review initially looks at what is meant by team building, the necessary conditions for its effectiveness, and offers descriptions of six principal approaches to developing effective teamworking:

team member selection
team building
team training
leadership training
team work re-design
organisational context interventions.

The HEA Multidisciplinary Team Workshop Programme is described and an analysis of the content and value of team-building workshops offered by LOTs is presented. Examples of good practice are given and the report concludes with a series of recommendations for future strategies for developing effective teamwork in primary health care.

# What is team building?

Given the growing use and importance of primary health care teams and the reality that teams in most organisations fail to perform optimally, what can be done to promote team effectiveness? This section answers this question by describing:

- the concept of team effectiveness
- basic requirements for team building
- key factors influencing team effectiveness
- the main types of team interventions employed in organisational settings
- research on the effectiveness of each model
- recommendations for practice.

Effectiveness refers to how well a team accomplishes its purpose (see the companion report on team effectiveness – West and Slater, 1996). It relates to a team's performance, including the quality and quantity of services it provides. However the term also refers to a team's ability to remain vital, innovate and grow, and to the wellbeing and development of team members. These factors all enable the team to sustain its performance and accomplish its mission over a period of time. Interventions therefore tend to focus on enhancing the effectiveness of teams in one or more of these domains. However, before attempting to enhance the effectiveness of interventions, four requirements should minimally be met, but are often not carefully considered by those offering interventions:

## 1. The use of teams must be appropriate

If there are no inderdependencies in the work of team members (i.e. they do not have to rely very much on one another to get the job done) or an individual can perform the task better, then developing a team is inappropriate. However, in the domain of primary health care many policy documents and research studies have indicated that teamwork in primary health care is valuable (West and Slater, 1996).

## 2. There is adequate management support

Considerable research has shown the importance of management support for teams (Tannenbaum, Salas and Cannon-Bowers, 1996; Guzzo and Shea, 1992) and that its absence can undermine team building to an extent which threatens the long-term stability of the team. This would include the commitment of community trust managers and of general practitioners.

## 3. The team receives adequate resources

Even well functioning teams are likely to fail if they lack the resources necessary to complete their task. As Hackman (1990) has indicated, team members need: adequate time to complete team tasks, access to information necessary for task completion, appropriate equipment, sufficient personnel and appropriate organisational structures and policies supporting teamwork.

### 4. The team's needs are correctly diagnosed

Different types of teams have different requirements for success and teams have different needs at different stages of their development. Consequently, no team intervention is likely to be effective in all situations. A team that lacks particular professional skills requires a rather different intervention from one which has communication problems or exhibits role conflict. Appropriate interventions cannot be chosen confidently before identifying a team's needs. Tannenbaum, Salas and Cannon-Bowers argue that some facilitators inappropriately rely on one predominant intervention for use with all teams, but correct diagnosis is critical for selecting the right intervention. Moreover, they argue that it is important for facilitators to be familiar with the full range of options available for enhancing team effectiveness.

# Types of team intervention

In this section, six principal types of team intervention are described, revealing the range of options available to those wishing to facilitate the development of teamwork in primary health care.

## 1. TEAM MEMBER SELECTION

Selection for teams refers to ways of identifying the best people to become team members. Although organisations tend to use quite sophisticated methods for selecting employees for individual jobs, they rarely use systematic methods for selecting people for teams. There is a number of reasons why selection interventions should improve team effectiveness. First, systematic selection methods can help identify people with greater skill levels. There is strong evidence that a team composed of skilled and motivated people will be more effective than other teams (Tziner, 1988). Selection interventions could improve effectiveness by increasing the professional or skill diversity of team members, thereby increasing the range of competencies in the group. There is clearly a value in considering the existing skill and experience mix of the team when selecting new or replacement team members.

Selection interventions will also help team performance by identifying those people who work best in a team environment. Working in teams requires people who are not only capable of performing their own task, but also possess knowledge, skills and attitudes (KSAs) that support their team. Skills such as supporting and building on the work of others, getting along with others and managing conflict are clearly important. Stevens and Campion (1994) have described some of the competency requirements for working in teams as follows:

### Conflict resolution KSAs

- Recognising and encouraging desirable, but discouraging undesirable, team conflict
- Employing appropriate conflict resolution strategies
- Using 'win-win' negotiation strategies

### Collaborative problem-solving KSAs

- Recognising situations requiring participative group problem-solving
- Overcoming obstacles to collaborative problem-solving

### Communication KSAs

- Communicating openly and supportively
- Listening non-evaluatively and actively

- Maximising consonance between verbal and non-verbal messages
- Engaging in ritual greetings and small talk, and recognising their importance

### Goal setting and performance management KSAs

- Establishing specific, challenging and accepted team goals
- Monitoring, evaluating and providing feedback on both overall team performance and individual team member performance

### Planning and task co-ordination KSAs

- Co-ordinating and synchronising activities and information between team members
- Helping to establish task and role expectations of individual team members, and ensure a proper balance of workloads in the team.

A related approach used by some LOTs in their team-building workshops is Belbin's concept of team roles (Belbin, 1993). Belbin uses a questionnaire to examine the consistency of team-related behaviours of individuals and argues for a mix of team role types (e.g. monitor-evaluator, resource investigator, completer-finisher). However, there is no convincing evidence that the questionnaire has satisfactory psychometric validity, or that team effectiveness is demonstrated by diversity of the team role types which Belbin identifies. Previous research suggests that competency-based approaches (focusing on knowledge, skills and abilities) are likely to be more effective methods of team member selection (Stevens and Campion, 1994).

## 2. TEAM BUILDING

Team building refers to a variety of interventions that typically focus on team interactions and processes. Team building is a type of process intervention aimed at helping individuals and groups examine and act upon their behaviour in team relationships. Although the general framework of team-building interventions may be established at the outset, the content of the intervention will, in part, be determined by discussions with all team members. Some team-building interventions focus on *role clarification*, some on *interpersonal relationships* or *conflict resolution* issues while others take more of a general *problem-solving approach* (Tannenbaum, Salas and Cannon-Bowers, 1996). *Team norms, attitudes, climate and power distribution* can be affected by team-building approaches. Many team processes, including *communication*, *decision-making* and *mutual role understanding*, are often direct targets of team-building interventions.

Team-building interventions often focus on increasing the *cohesiveness* of teams in order to improve team performance, based on the assumption that increasing team cohesion will lead to better team performance. A recent review of the literature examining the relationship between *cohesiveness and team performance* has indeed demonstrated the existence of a small, but significant relationship. However, this review (Mullen and Copper, 1993) also indicated that it was good team performance which produced cohesiveness rather than vice versa. This suggests that building cohesiveness in teams will not necessarily have any direct impact upon team performance, whereas improving team performance is likely to have an impact upon team cohesiveness.

Conflict can adversely affect cohesiveness and reduce team effectiveness. However, avoiding conflict is not a solution; some conflict is inevitable and indeed is desirable (Pascale, 1990; West, 1994). *Conflict resolution* is potentially an important element of team-building interventions since constructive conflict can lead to improved team performance and innovation (West, 1996). However, facilitators often avoid this topic since it arouses their own anxieties about dealing with conflict in team-building events.

Several reviews have examined the efficacy of team-building interventions (DeMeuse and Liebowitz, 1981; Sundstrom, DeMeuse and Futrell, 1990; Tannenbaum, Beard and Salas, 1992; Guzzo and Shea, 1992). They suggest that no one team-building method consistently works better than others. *The cumulative evidence suggests that while team-building interventions can have a positive impact on individual perceptions and attitudes, there is less support for any impact upon team performance.* Team performance is a function of many factors, some of which are well beyond the scope of most team-building interventions and therefore it may be optimistic to assume that one workshop will radically affect team performance. This evidence should enable LOTs, and others involved in team building in this area, to have realistic expectations about what a team-building intervention can accomplish. It may be unrealistic to rely on team building as the sole mechanism for improving team performance. Instead team building should best be considered as part of a larger improvement strategy augmented by other interventions dictated by the specific needs of the team – such as bringing about changes in the organisational structure of primary health care.

Overall research strongly suggests that team-building interventions that help clarify *team and individual goals* should enhance team effectiveness (Guzzo and Shea, 1992).

## 3. TEAM TRAINING

Team training is a set of instructional strategies and tools aimed at enhancing teamwork, knowledge, skills, processes and performance. Team training is a systematic effort to facilitate the development of team members' knowledge, skills and attitudes such as co-ordination, communication and decision-making. For example under the conditions of high workload, time pressure and other kinds of stress which most primary health care teams experience at some time, effective co-ordination of team members' work is critical if they are to perform effectively.

Recently, Cannon-Bowers, Salas and Converse (1993) have argued that effective team performance will only occur if team members have a *shared understanding* of the task, their team colleagues' roles and expertise, as well as the context (e.g. health needs of the local population) in which they operate. Moreover, team members need to have *accurate expectations* of their team colleagues, the task demands and the environment in which they operate. It is the ability to anticipate team members' professional behaviour that enables teams to co-ordinate effectively. One team training technique designed to achieve this is *cross-training*. Team members are cross-trained on team colleagues' tasks in order to help them be clearer about the structure of the team and the task, the inter-relationships among team members' positions, and the roles and responsibility of each team member. This improves team performance by enhancing *common task and team expectations*.

A second strategy is *team co-ordination training*. This is a strategy designed to enhance *teamwork skills*, *team processes* and *communication* including *decision-making*, *assertiveness*, *team leadership*, *adaptability* and *planning*. The objectives of the training are to demonstrate effective and ineffective teamwork skills and create opportunities to practise them. A variety of methods are used to fulfil these training objectives including lectures, video demonstrations, role playing and simulations. Teamwork is promoted by providing relevant information about team members' tasks and responsibilities; demonstrating effective and ineffective teamwork behaviour; and creating opportunities to practise (by role playing, simulation on the job) and providing feedback on critical aspects of team functioning.

Team meetings and decision-making are centrally important for effective team functioning. Future interventions could particularly benefit from the design and development of team training interventions which allow team members to practise managing meetings, and using task relevant information such as practice profiles or health needs analysis for effective team decision-making.

## 4. LEADERSHIP TRAINING

Leadership training refers to methods of enhancing a team leader's capabilities. Recently team leaders in many organisations have been required to change from the traditional supervisory role to that of a facilitator or coach (Tannenbaum, Salas and Cannon-Bowers, 1996). The team leader's relationship with team members in this approach is less hierarchical and autocratic and more collaborative, and involves removing obstacles to team performance, facilitating team processes and helping team members build their competencies. Indeed, the concept of teamwork in modern complex organisations is one which strongly emphasises autonomy and devolved responsibility (Cordery, 1996).

Within primary health care, the issue of team leadership remains ambiguous and uncertain because of the diverse lines of management into primary health care teams (West, 1996). However, there is much evidence that suggests team leaders have considerable influence on team performance (Brewer, Wilson and Beck, 1994). Team leaders bring to teams their individual expertise as well as feedback, coaching and influencing skills. In even the most democratic teams, team leaders often have the greatest influence of any team member in defining work structure and influencing team climate through their leadership style. Moreover, they are influential in determining team processes such as communication, decision-making and problem-solving. This is evidenced by the resultant changes in team processes when leadership changes occur. For these reasons interventions that enhance the team leader's effectiveness will often improve team performance. There are many methods of promoting better team leadership including *leadership training, coaching* and *360° feedback.* (The 360° feedback method involves everyone in the team giving all other team members feedback on their performance (Tannenbaum, Salas and Cannon-Bowers, 1996; Yukl and Vanfleet, 1992).)

## 5. TEAM WORK RE-DESIGN

Another category of team interventions is used to modify or restructure the way work is performed – how work flows through a team, how it is assigned, how the task is organised and the amount of flexibility and autonomy team members have in performing tasks and making decisions. One of the most prevalent restructuring approaches is referred to as *process re-engineering*. This method involved the diagnosis and modification of work and information flow in an attempt to reduce inefficiencies, streamline operations and improve performance (e.g. introducing nurse triage for requests for home visits or introducing a nurse practitioner role in the team). Re-engineering has been applied extensively throughout many organisations, though not always specifically targeting team tasks and performance. Another approach to work re-design is increasing *team autonomy* and *participation in decision-making*. There is evidence that greater participation in work decisions can increase performance and productivity (Cotton *et al.*, 1988; Pearson, 1987). Consequently, many organisations have increased the extent to which teams control work-related decisions. Examples of this are seen in the application of self-managing, semi-autonomous or autonomous work groups (Cordery, 1996).

A number of interventions encourage greater fluidity and *role flexibility* in team structure (Nahavandi and Aranda, 1994) so that roles overlap and change, as required by the changing and demanding nature of the work. The rationale behind this is that patient needs are changing rapidly, so teams must have greater flexibility to respond quickly. Traditional team structures and rigid professional identities, with carefully delineated boundaries between jobs, produce teams which are less capable of responding to rapid change.

## 6. ORGANISATIONAL CONTEXT INTERVENTIONS

Considerable research evidence indicates that organisational context plays a powerful role in influencing team effectiveness. Organisations influence team effectiveness to the extent that they provide:

- education for teamwork
- rewards for teams (as opposed to individuals)
- adequate resource for teams
- relevant information
- support for teamworking
- clear management
- clear objectives
- feedback on team performance.

Another approach to developing team effectiveness therefore is to see team building as a secondary strategy which should only be undertaken after contextual and structural issues have been addressed. In the case of primary health care teams, this orientation would argue for:

- resolving the anomalous independent contractor status of GPs vis-à-vis other professionals in the team
- rationalising the reward system so that teams receive bonuses for good performance rather than one professional in the team
- creating a consistent and single line of management into primary health care teams
- ensuring adequate training for teamworking at the individual as well as at the team level
- enabling teams to develop clear strategies for meeting health care needs of their local populations
- providing clear and accurate feedback on team performance
- providing assistance for developing teamwork
- determining who will lead primary health care teams.

These approaches have been used in private sector organisations but have not been developed within the primary health care context, despite the particular organisational difficulties faced by teams in this context.

These are some of the principal approaches to building effective teamwork employed in organisational settings. Their use depends upon the particular needs of teams and the context in which the teams operate. Their description illustrates the diversity of intervention types and the breadth of interventions potentially available to those wishing to build more effective teamwork in primary health care. The remaining sections of this review provide an overview of the approaches to team building adopted by LOTs and other groups and illustrate the enormous influence the Multidisciplinary Team Workshop Programme has had on primary health care teams in the UK.

# The HEA Multidisciplinary Team Workshop Programme

In 1987 the HEA initiated a major national strategy for developing primary health care team working (Spratley, 1989) which has had an enormous impact upon primary health care and professional development. The primary health care team Multidisciplinary Team Workshop (MDTW) Programme was initiated in order to promote health education and disease prevention on a national scale. The HEA MDTW Programme model was based on a number of principles:

- Teams should be centred or based on general practices
- The workshop should be multidisciplinary
- All primary health care workers should have the opportunity to participate in a mutual learning experience
- Team members should have the opportunity to learn to work together to achieve a common goal
- Individuals should be respected for their skills and experience and their roles in planning should reflect this
- The workshop should be sensitive to the needs and problems of the participants
- Each team should develop its own style of working with no predetermined leader and with minimal interference from the workshop facilitators
- Each team should start from its own baseline and set its own planning objectives
- Each team should work at its own pace
- Each team should be free to choose its own topic or area of work
- Each team should be free to choose a strategy to adopt
- Each team should be encouraged to consider the difficulties that might arise in putting forward plans for policy and organisational changes to colleagues.

The first of the workshops was held in 1987 and the success of the early workshops led to extensive development of the programme. The problems of disseminating the successful model stimulated an initiative to develop a nationwide system of local organising teams (LOTs) which took responsibility for applying the model in their areas. The aims of the MDTW Programme are:

- To promote health and reduce ill health and disability in the population, while enhancing where possible the quality of life
- To encourage understanding of the roles, skills and experience of each person in the primary health care team
- To encourage and stimulate better communication in teamwork
- To develop plans and organisational changes that support disease prevention and health promotion
- To provide an opportunity for reflection on the present organisation of teamwork, communication, health education and disease prevention activities and to consider how these might be improved
- To encourage the recognition of resources within the community
- To encourage the development of mutual support mechanisms.

The programme has been enormously successful and the model has been employed with minor variations by LOTs throughout the country.

The MDTW Programme was evaluated after two years (Spratley, 1989) and a number of beneficial outcomes were identified, particularly in the areas of communication and teamwork. Spratley observed the following outcomes:

- improvement of teamworking skills
- enhanced understanding of team roles
- improved multidisciplinary working
- increased understanding of health promotion
- the development of better practice information
- development of action plans
- reviews of practice organisation
- identification of resource requirements
- sharing of knowledge and experience between teams
- identification of professional development needs.

However, the evaluation relied largely on immediate post-intervention self-reports from participants and such reports exhibit a strong halo effect which is likely to over-emphasise the true impact of interventions. As observed earlier, team-building interventions tend to have reliably positive impacts upon attitudes and perceptions of team members, but little impact on team performance.

The HEA MDTW Programme has had a major influence throughout the country, partly because of the development of excellent materials to support LOTs and others concerned to develop teamwork in primary health care and also because of the enormous enthusiasm that LOT members and primary health care team members have shown for the strategy. This commitment and enthusiasm is demonstrated in the following section where LOT members' descriptions of the MDTW Programme are presented.

# LOT representatives' descriptions of their team-building exercises

Questionnaires were sent to representatives of 70 LOTs, seeking information about the approach to team building they employed in their work with multidisciplinary teams in primary health care. Questions covered the methods used in team-building workshops, the content of the team-building workshops, the attendees, the underlying principles and the effectiveness of the workshops (see Appendix B for the content of the questionnaire). Thirty-two responses were received.

## MODELS, METHODS AND CONTENT

LOT members were asked to describe the overall aims of the team-building workshops, and the main elements of those workshops. Most frequently cited aims were as follows:

- team building
- improving teamworking
- improving health promotion
- improving communication
- increasing understanding and respect amongst professionals
- clarifying roles and skills.

Main elements of the team-building workshop most frequently mentioned were:

- role clarification
- team objectives and common goals
- action planning
- skills audit.

Those less frequently mentioned were:

- health needs analysis
- power and control
- health promotion
- organisational audit.

LOT representatives were then asked the extent to which they covered each of 20 specified areas in their team-building workshops such as team objectives, health needs assessment, health promotion, role clarification, shared decision-making. A full list of the areas they were asked to judge is included in the questionnaire reproduced in Appendix B. LOT members were asked to indicate the extent to which they covered the areas on a scale ranging from '*not at all*' through '*little*', '*moderately*', '*quite substantially*' to '*very substantially*'. The most frequently mentioned areas covered in the LOT team-building workshops were, in order of frequency, as follows:

- getting to know one another as people
- communication
- developing mutual role understanding
- team collaboration
- role clarification
- relationships between professionals
- building cohesion.

Least frequently mentioned areas were:

- disease prevention
- relationships with patients
- protocol development
- health needs assessment
- innovations in practice
- health promotion.

This pattern of responses reveals a consistent orientation in these team-building workshops towards building cohesive relationships between team members rather than addressing task-related issues such as health needs assessment, health promotion, relationships with patients and disease prevention. Indeed, disease prevention was the second least frequently covered area. Team meetings, shared decision-making and team objectives were also infrequently covered. These latter three represent fundamental elements of team processes in terms of improving team functioning. The least frequently addressed areas represent specific task-related issues. It seems that the most common model of team building employed by LOTs is what has been called a 'human relations' process model in preference to team task design approaches. The human relations model was particularly dominant between the 1960s and 1980s but theory and research have indicated that improving team functioning on tasks is likely to promote team cohesion whereas building team cohesiveness may have little impact on team effectiveness (Guzzo and Shea, 1992; Mullen and Copper, 1994).

LOT representatives were also asked to indicate the extent to which they used syndicate or small group exercises, lectures or other forms of activity in the team-building workshops. Responses indicated that, in most, two-thirds of the time was taken up by syndicate or small group work and one-third by lectures or other activities. Typical content areas included role clarification, theory of team building, team tasks of team's own choosing, practice plans, managing change, team-building exercises, communication exercises and considerable time spent on action planning. Most LOTs encouraged teams to work on developing action plans in relation to a specific objective concerned either with team processes or health care. Other areas, less frequently covered, included the new structure of the NHS, health needs assessment, managing change, bereavement, assertiveness, self-awareness and even a ceilidh and various games.

## ATTENDANCE AT WORKSHOPS

LOT members indicated that on average 42 per cent of primary health care teams in their areas had taken part in the team-building workshops, with typically around 35 people in each workshop. Some comments about these figures are noteworthy. In the first place, it is a testament to the enormous enthusiasm and marketing ability of LOT members that they have encouraged nearly half of the teams in their areas to participate in at least one team-building workshop. On the other hand, with 35 people attending the amount of attention and individual coaching that can be given to teams is clearly very limited. Most team training and team-building exercises outside the NHS would involve groups no larger than 15–20 people, in order that facilitators can provide close coaching for teams. The strategy adopted by LOTs is understandable given the limitations on time and resources, a topic which we will return to later. Moreover, some LOT members report a lack of confidence in coaching teams and uncertainty about their own expertise and competence in developing primary health care teamwork. Many referred to their lack of theoretical knowledge of evidence-based approaches to developing effective teamwork.

When asked who typically attends the workshop sessions, the responses of LOT representatives revealed that in only a minority of cases did the whole practice team, plus other community professionals attend the workshops. Most usual was for some members of the practice team, plus some community nurses to attend – in effect, a sub-sample of the primary health care team. On average, five teams were represented at each workshop. It was usual across almost all the LOTs for all the principal primary health care professionals to be represented, i.e. GPs, health visitors, district nurses, practice nurses, administrators, receptionists and practice managers. However, in one case the LOT made it a condition of attendance that at least one GP attended. In another LOT no community staff were invited and in still another the approach was to invite uni-professional groups. Typically, around 40 per cent of the practice team attended team-building workshops, a figure which many LOT team members felt was too low.

## THE VENUE

The team-building workshops usually lasted for two or two-and-a-half days and were generally residential. This was by far and away the most common model employed in team-building workshops. In a small number of cases the workshops lasted for only a day or half a day. Most of the team-building events were completed in one session, but short follow-up sessions with many teams enabled some spread of the team-building activities to occur. There was a fairly equal split between workshops held at weekdays or at weekends, and almost all LOTs conducted their team-building workshops in hotels. Only two conducted them within practice settings. Other settings used were conference centres, colleges of education and universities. Most LOTs provided some follow-up after the workshops, which usually consisted of a visit or telephone call to determine whether action planning at the workshops had been implemented. Input to the workshops was provided predominantly by LOT members. This is noteworthy given the frequently stated insecurity that LOT members voiced about their knowledge of theoretical approaches and research evidence about team-based working. Outside lecturers were brought in by less than half of the LOTs. Other inputs were sought from chief executives and management consultants.

## EFFECTIVENESS OF TEAM-BUILDING WORKSHOPS

LOT members were asked which were the most effective and ineffective components of the team-building workshops they provided and why.
Effective elements identified were:

- group work on tasks
- practice planning

- work on issues of practices' own choosing (generally, primary health care teams were asked to identify one issue which they wished to address during the team-building workshops and develop a relevant action plan. This was the most emphasised activity in many team-building workshops and enabled teams to make useful progress and to explore working as a team)
- role definition
- team building
- the social aspects of the events
- protected time away from work enabling primary health care team members to get to know each other.

Least effective elements were identified as:

- limited representation of teams at the workshops, making it difficult to implement the action plans back in practices
- gaining commitment, especially from GPs
- low uptake by primary health care teams
- formal inputs and keynote addresses
- ineffective follow-up activity
- action plans not being implemented by teams
- not being able to provide hard evidence of improvements in primary health care team functioning.

When asked in what ways the team-building workshops could be improved significantly, the most frequently mentioned elements were:

- better pre-workshop planning and more time with teams for diagnosis
- better uptake
- involving the whole primary health care team
- organising more advanced development workshops for those primary health care teams which had made progress
- models of team building which could be appropriately applied to different types of teams
- more cash, time, support and training for LOTs in order that they could do an even more professional job
- measurable objectives, so enabling better evaluation
- post-workshop support, particularly improving the follow-up that LOTs provided.

Respondents to the questionnaire were asked to indicate the extent to which they felt that investment in team building produced more efficient and effective health services on a scale ranging from 'very limited results' through 'moderate results', to 'quite good results', 'very good results' and 'outstanding results'. Forty-eight per cent indicated very good results, 25 per cent indicated quite good results and 25 per cent indicated moderate results. LOT member comments included the following:

'The outcomes depend on the commitment and motivation of participants.'
'Teams need to want to work as a team.'
'LOTs need training and time-out as a team to keep their direction.'
'Ideally primary health care teams should be offered continuous support.'
'LOT members are extremely busy and have no time, financial or clerical support or recognition for the valuable work that they do.'

Finally, LOT members were asked what would be the key demands on primary health care teams in the future. Most mentioned the shift from secondary to primary care with a consequent increase in demands on primary health care services. Others mentioned:

- patient expectations
- the need to plan and organise better to cope with pressures
- changes in demands
- managing change
- increasing workload
- more professional groups involved in primary health care
- developing GP fundholder purchasing plans
- staff appraisal and development
- the need to develop practice and community profiles
- the devolution of managerial and ethical accountability to primary health care members.

It was striking that, in general, these strategic issues identified by LOT members were very rarely addressed as part of the team-building workshops.

The lessons to be learned from the responses to the questionnaire are numerous. The first is that the workshops to which primary health care teams are exposed through the Health Education Authority programme are a very helpful way of developing primary health care professionals' awareness of teamworking. The dedication of LOT members and primary health care team members in participating in the programmes is also most impressive. The main focus of many workshops appears to be on building cohesion (which has only limited impacts upon team effectiveness). On the other hand, a variety of task-related issues and particularly the development of strategic approaches to primary health care tend to be neglected. LOT members also report feeling inadequately trained and lacking knowledge about theories and research evidence relating to team functioning and team effectiveness. They repeatedly emphasised the lack of resources and support to function effectively as organising teams. If the concepts of effective teamwork discussed earlier in this and the companion report (West and Slater, 1996) were applied to LOT teams, we would predict limited team effectiveness, precisely because they often lack appropriate organisational support.

# Evaluation of workshops by LOTs

LOT representatives were asked to describe how they evaluated the team-building workshops. The vast majority relied on participants' ratings via questionnaires which covered ratings of content, venues, speakers, and the value of specific workshop sessions. Other approaches involved an assessment of the extent to which team action plans were implemented and whether the objectives of attendees were achieved. All but two of the LOTs used non-standardised, unvalidated questionnaires to assess the extent to which change resulted from the team-building workshops. Most of the questionnaires were self-designed and consisted of self-report on unvalidated instruments. The only exceptions were the use by two LOTs of the Team Climate Inventory (Anderson and West, 1994), which examines clarity of team objectives, levels of participation, task orientation, support for innovation, mutual role understanding and appropriate mutual skill use in primary health care teams.

Two-thirds of the LOTs evaluated the team-building workshops only after the event while one-third used instruments both before and after to measure change in team member perceptions. The vast majority of evaluations were conducted immediately after the workshops (i.e. two-thirds). One-third also evaluated the team-building workshops six months later though this was usually in the form of a visit or telephone call to the practice to determine the extent to which the action plan had been implemented.

Thus, in general, the evaluation of the LOT workshops has been carried out carefully by LOT teams. There has been a clear commitment by almost all LOT teams to evaluate the content of the workshops and to gather participants' reactions to their impact. Moreover, many have adopted a long-term follow-up strategy for evaluating outcomes, often visiting the teams to determine how effectively they had implemented their action plans. This degree of commitment to evaluation of interventions is testament to the professionalism of LOTs.

However, the evaluation of the workshops has been based largely on self-report using instruments of unknown validity and reliability. Consequently, it is difficult to evaluate their true impact. Research into the effectiveness of team building has repeatedly demonstrated positive halo effects immediately following interventions. In other words, those participating in interventions tend to evaluate them very positively immediately after the workshops (which is when most LOT evaluations took place). However, such self-report measures rarely provide an indication of the impact of interventions upon team performance.

Reviews of research into team building reveal that they generally tend to have a positive impact upon perceptions and attitudes of team members towards one another, but little impact upon the effectiveness of the team in its performance (Woodman and Sherwood, 1980; DeMeuse and Liebowitz, 1981; Liebowitz and DeMeuse, 1982; Tannenbaum, Beard and Salas, 1992; Guzzo and Shea, 1992; Tannenbaum, Salas and Cannon-Bowers (1996), though for an important exception see Pritchard, 1991).

However, one careful study of the effect of the LOT team-building workshops has been carried out by Poulton (1995). She adopted a pre- and post-intervention design, but without equivalent control groups. Primary health care teams intending to attend

LOT workshops were identified and requested to complete self-report questionnaires before and three months after the workshops. All members of the primary health care team were asked to complete questionnaires and not simply those attending the LOT workshops. Members of 39 primary health care teams completed the questionnaires. Poulton used the Team Climate Inventory (Anderson and West, 1994), a validated measure of team functioning which examines four areas:

- clarity of team objectives
- team participation
- task orientation
- support for innovation.

In addition, Poulton employed scales measuring mutual role understanding, appropriate skill use and valuing of professionals within the primary health care team. Comparisons of pre- and post-workshop scores revealed a significant increase in levels of participation, task orientation, clarity of team objectives, understanding of others' team roles and appropriate skill use. Those who attended the team workshops rated their teams significantly higher post-workshops than non-participants. These findings suggest that the team workshops do have an impact upon the quality of team functioning within teams, though this effect is seen as more marked by those who attend the workshops than those who do not.

Indeed one concern raised by LOT representatives relates to the potential impact of a sub-team engaging in team development activities and then returning to the wider team to disseminate the results of their work. Boss and McConkie (1981) have drawn attention to such problems and recommend that methods be developed to facilitate team member re-entry into the team following interventions.

Overall, responses of LOT members reveal a pattern of dedicated and substantial activity across the country which has changed professionals' views of teamworking in general, and their own team's functioning specifically. This is an excellent basis for the continued development of teamworking in primary care.

# Examples of good practice

In this section we describe seven examples of team building and team development in primary health care which offer alternatives to the standard workshop model employed by many LOTs. Although the model used by LOTs is clearly effective in changing attitudes and perceptions of people within teams, these additional examples of good practice are described because they offer complementary or more advanced approaches to developing team-based working within primary health care. It is not intended to describe all the many examples of good practice occurring around the country, but merely to offer representative examples of different approaches.

## 1. PRIMARY HEALTH CARE TEAM DEVELOPMENT PROGRAMME – UNITED HEALTH COMMISSION

The United Health Commission in South Humberside has constructed a programme comprising five modular projects which interlink to produce a Primary Health Care Team Development Programme of considerable substance. The five modules cover:

- mental health strategy
- organisational audit
- shared-care seminars
- primary health care team workshops
- practice-based health needs assessment.

The mental health strategy module aims to improve the primary health care teams' ability to recognise common psychological conditions and to develop a shared care strategy between the acute and primary sectors. The module is designed to develop guidelines and protocols for primary health care teams; to improve the health and social functioning of mentally ill people; to reduce the overall suicide rate by 15 per cent by the year 2000; and to reduce the suicide rate of severely mentally ill people by 33 per cent by the year 2000.

The second module – organisational audit – aims to assist practices in developing their own quality standards for the way their services are organised. This module focuses on administrative structures and procedures which are required to support high quality patient care. The organisational audit enables practices to set standards for organisational functioning and to evaluate their performance against those standards.

The third component, shared care seminars, aims to build alliances between those working in primary and secondary care and produces mutually agreed protocols for shared responsibility in the treatment of conditions such as diabetes, asthma or heart disease.

The primary health care team workshops provide teams with time-out away from general practice and enable team members to concentrate on a topic of their choice (such as heart disease). The commission brings teams together, offers lectures and facilitates teams in devising a project which can be taken forward in the practice.

The final component offers practice profiling for primary health care teams in order that they can gain an overview of the health needs in their areas. It assists the primary health care team in developing a strategy for responding to needs in the area. It employs a combination of epidemiology, local needs assessment and planning in order to support the development of strategic approaches to the delivery of primary health care by the whole team.

The principal value of the United Health Commission approach resides in its combination of a number of components for organisational change, making it more likely to generate improvements in primary health care. Of course such a programme was also dependent on having sufficient expertise to feed into the programme and sufficient financial resourcing to enable primary health care teams to attend given the difficulties of teams getting cover and the costs of running workshops.

## 2. TEAM CARE VALLEYS INITIATIVE

The Team Care Valleys (TCV) Initiative in South Wales was launched in October 1990 and ended in August 1993. As a unit of University of Wales College of Medicine, funded by the Welsh Office, TCV draws on the multidisciplinary knowledge and skills of a team of general practitioners, nurses, health visitors, lecturers in practice management and social scientists.

The overall aim of the project was to help develop primary health care services within South Wales Valleys communities. Activities were focused on general practice, community nurses, health visitors and other health care workers in the area and aimed at promoting the positive benefits of multi- and interdisciplinary teamworking in primary care. This was achieved through provision of education and training programmes, facilitating research, establishing a practice advisory service and other practical measures which helped sustain and complement the commitment of all those involved in primary care throughout the area. The objectives of the programme were to:

- establish research projects which would explore and evaluate new ways of providing primary health care
- provide continuing professional education and training programmes of direct operational value
- provide support to enable innovation in provision of primary health care
- provide a resource of professional expertise to assist primary health care practitioners in the pursuit of a quality service
- establish an effective interface with key organisations and users in primary health care
- research, evaluate and promote the positive benefits of primary health care teamworking
- constructively develop teamworking through training and other associated practical measures
- provide opportunities for TCV staff to develop skills, knowledge and expertise through professional staff development plans.

The programme represents the kind of comprehensive and strategic approach to the management of organisational change which has been demonstrated to be more effective than piecemeal single-issue approaches (Guzzo, 1996). The advantage of this type of an approach, which has a number of strands, is that it is more likely to achieve real change in primary health care than single workshops, focused on single issues. Of course, such an initiative requires high levels of expertise, considerable financial resources, and the willing involvement of primary health care teams.

## 3. MULTIDISCIPLINARY AUDIT

At the Eli Lilly National Clinical Audit Centre, University of Leicester, a sophisticated approach to the facilitation of multi-professional clinical audit in primary health care teams has been developed. The programme aims to apply total quality management principles in order to:

- help primary health care teams maximise resources
- clarify teams' aims and objectives
- create improvement opportunities
- develop management strategies to achieve those objectives
- develop team skills within the primary health care team
- create a working environment where clinical audit becomes second nature.

The methodology incorporates a number of stages. First, a topic for audit is selected by a primary health care team. Teams are asked to identify particular problems in care which they select for audit and then to identify the standards that they would aim to achieve in a particular domain such as the care of diabetes. The team then collectively set standards, assess current levels of performance and determine action plans designed to enable them to achieve the standards set. After the implementation of their action plan, team performance is evaluated against the set standards and new action plans are drawn up. The audit cycle therefore involves:

- choosing a topic or identifying a problem
- setting target standards
- observing practice
- comparing performance with targets
- implementing change
- again setting targets and standards.

An example of a target standard in relation to *patient access to primary health care services* would be the offer of routine appointments within three working days. The aim might then be that the criterion is met for 90 per cent of patients. In relation to the criterion, *penicillin allergy to be marked on the front of patient notes*, the standard might be that this must apply to 100 per cent of patients. The group at the Eli Lilly National Clinical Audit Centre have incorporated a number of models from other organisational settings to facilitate the process. For example, they use cause-and-effect diagrams, total quality management concepts, flowcharts, measures of customer satisfaction (by patient satisfaction questionnaires) and teamworking exercises widely used in commercial organisational settings.

The main advantage of the approach is that it provides a highly structured and objective method for improving effectiveness in defined areas. It requires skilled facilitators, although the Eli Lilley National Clinical Audit Centre has produced excellent support material for facilitators, in the form of videos and written information. Clearly, the resource implications are considerable given the required expertise of the facilitator and the continuing support needed for teams (at least initially). Nevertheless, this represents a very useful programme for developing primary health care effectiveness in specific disease areas. Overall it lacks the strategic orientation to primary health care team working incorporated in other approaches.

Thus, the means of developing a co-ordinated team approach to decision-making, objective setting and strategy development for the delivery of primary health care in a locality on a continuing basis is not directly addressed by this programme.

## 4. TEAM BUILDING IN PRIMARY CARE – CHESHIRE COMMUNITY HEALTH

The approach adopted by the Cheshire Community Health Care Trust to team building in primary care is underpinned by three principles. The first is that team-building processes should be based on information derived from literature and research where possible, i.e. they believe it is essential to establish a broad knowledge base about team development. The second is that facilitators must have expertise in working with teams and be knowledgeable about group development. The third requirement is for facilitators who have knowledge about the primary health care context and who are aware of the constraints, politics, systems, structures and rules in that domain:

> The process of team development is thus a complex one which cannot be left to chance. It must be facilitated in a careful and skilful manner if it is to be a positive experience. Mindful of some of our own somewhat dubious experiences of team building, this was a further reason for enlisting the expertise of an external facilitator. (Knapman *et al.*, 1995, p. 18)

The approach to team building used by the Cheshire model involves defining *the concept of team*, exploring common *teamwork problems* and the *consequences of poor teamwork*, as well as the essential *components for effective teamwork*. The facilitation incorporates input on *ground rules for team building*, *stages of team development* and *models of adult learning and organisational change*.

This group explicitly articulates the view that the role of team-builder requires adequate knowledge and skill to discharge the role competently and ethically, a view which we found rarely expressed by those involved in team building in primary health care. Given that any development team process has potential difficulties such as intra or inter-personal conflicts as well as possible detrimental impacts upon role functioning, the ethical implications of interventions are considerable. However these are rarely referred to in the literature and materials produced by those involved in developing team building in primary health care. One particular advantage of the approach described by Knapman and colleagues is that it adopts a clear perspective on the need for team building to be based upon well-substantiated theoretical approaches and for facilitation, grounded in expertise in the management of group development and group dynamics.

One disadvantage of this approach is that it adopts a largely 'single issue' approach to team building, in that the teams involved in the programme usually address one area of the team's activities in developing an action plan. A strategic approach to developing primary health care in a locality involving all of the professionals in formulating strategy is neglected.

## 5. THE MICROPURCHASING PROJECT – NORTHERN AND YORKSHIRE REGION

The Northern and Yorkshire Region model of team building – Micropurchasing Project – had five guiding principles:

*To identify strategic objectives* for primary health care teams, based on health needs analysis. This requires a primary health care team to use a variety of data sources, including their own experience, to identify and prioritise the health needs of their local population.

*Devolution of management* – The project encouraged the devolution of management down to primary care team level by shifting the emphasis of the role of nurse managers from directing and monitoring to supporting and facilitating. Where possible, budgets were devolved down to nursing and general practice teams in order that teams could make autonomous decisions about the allocation of resources. There was also an attempt to devolve responsibility for decisions from general practitioners to others in the team where appropriate.

*Allocation of resources* – Primary health care team members were encouraged to audit their existing skills and resources and to determine where it was possible to reallocate these resources to respond to the prioritised health care needs of the local population. For example, in one team nurses undertook telephone triage in order to determine whether GP visits, nursing home visits or surgery appointments were the most appropriate medium for dealing with patient issues.

*Professional growth and development and clinical supervision* – If required skills did not exist within the team to meet prioritised health needs adequately, new members were recruited or existing members received training. The extent of new training across all teams involved in the project was considerable and professional growth and development was reportedly a widespread and valued consequence of the programme. Clinical supervision was also emphasised since team members took on new tasks as a consequence of the initiative. The models of clinical supervision were generally facilitative supportive models with professionals often providing mutual clinical supervision sessions in order to ensure best practice and appropriate reflection on practice.

*Evaluation* – The programme was evaluated using standardised instruments which examined team functioning (Anderson and West, 1994) in four areas: clarity of team objectives, participation (interaction, information sharing and influence over decision-making), task orientation and support for innovation. Significant improvement along all four dimensions of the questionnaire occurred for all nine teams which participated during the 12-month life of the project.

The intervention was also evaluated using a 23-item questionnaire which measured the effectiveness of primary health care teamwork along four dimensions:

- quality of patient care
- organisational effectiveness
- team development
- patient issues.

The initiative indicated significant improvement along all four dimensions. This is one of the few projects to use objective indicators of both team functioning and team outcomes as a result of team building in primary health care (West, Poulton and Hardy, 1994).

The Micropurchasing Project was facilitated by expert facilitators over a period of one year and involved a considerable amount of resource input. However, the approach encouraged team members to develop strategies for addressing the health needs of local populations, and encouraged all team members to be continually involved in team decision-making about how those health needs might best be met and how the resources available to the team might best be allocated.

## 6. THE KING'S FUND ORGANISATION AUDIT (KFOA)

The KFOA is aimed at improving the quality of health care by the application of organisational standards and a system of peer review, not just in primary health care, but in other health care settings. The organisational audit programme has been applied in 200 acute NHS and private hospitals in the UK. In January 1994 organisational audit for primary health care was launched and the programme has been applied to more than 60 health centres and GP practices across the UK.

Organisational audit involves an audit of the whole primary health care organisation based on a framework of standards and criteria for evaluating systems for the delivery of health care. Compliance with those standards is assessed by a team of senior health care professionals, who themselves have had a period of training and preparation. The underlying principle is that there is a relationship between organisational efficiency and effectiveness and good patient care. Thus, the rationale is that organisations have to be clear about their purpose, employees have to be committed to that purpose, and that structures and processes across the organisation should exist to achieve this purpose. As a result, clinical and non-clinical objectives are more likely to be achieved. Key areas examined include patients' rights, organisational arrangements, communication, staff development and education, health and safety and quality of care. There are three key stages:

- Using the organisational audit manual the primary health care team works with the standards and criteria set. A co-ordinator is appointed to lead the process and a steering group is appointed to facilitate the effectiveness of the audit process. Initial baseline measurements of performance against the standards and criteria are made.
- An independent team of senior health professionals undertakes a peer review survey of the performance of the primary health care team against the standards and criteria outlined in the organisational audit manual. The survey involves the documentation review, meetings with staff and visits to observe the facilities and services. The survey lasts about one-and-a-half days.
- The staff are verbally debriefed at the end of the survey and a detailed written report is submitted 6 to 8 weeks later. This provides a comprehensive evaluation of the effectiveness of the primary health care team. The report includes recommendations for change, as well as indications of good practice. As a result of this analysis it is possible for the team to identify areas in which change is required and to develop appropriate strategies to do so.

This intervention appears to be an effective way of diagnosing the work of a primary health care team and represents an example of good practice at the first stage of team development. Many primary health care teams embark on programmes of team building which may well not be suitable for them and which may well not address, what are in reality, the priority issues for the team if they are to best serve the needs of their local populations. KFOA offers a standardised way of approaching self-examination as an organisation which can identify gaps between existing and ideal good practice in organisational functioning.

The limitations of the approach are that a facilitator is required who can then help the team translate the recommendations into practice. The other potential weakness of KFOA, if it is used in isolation, is that no system for addressing the health care needs in the external environment is described. Thus while it is excellent to audit existing internal organisational practice, it does not appear to address the match between the primary health care organisation and its environment. Nevertheless, this example clearly represents an unusual and useful approach to the development of primary health care teamwork.

## 7. PRIMARY CARE TEAM DEVELOPMENT – DORSET HEALTH

Dorset Health Initiative aims to enhance the quality of primary care by:

- establishing new ways of working for primary health teams
- enabling the primary health care team to move from patient co-ordination to multi-professional health care management
- promoting systematic implementation of health care policies
- identifying critical success factors in team development.

The overall programme is underpinned by total quality management requirements:

- clear leadership (by GP partners and practice managers)
- all primary care team members involved
- covers clinical, administrative and organisational themes
- regular means for team discussions of primary health care issues
- the primary health care team as a whole discusses mission and objectives/targets
- patients are involved in the process and means of measuring patient satisfaction are developed
- staff development programme
- development of a practice business plan.

The initiative begins with an analysis of practices in terms of basic facts such as:

- team size
- practice organisation, e.g. consulting times, clinics, appointment times
- liaison and teamworking
- what meetings are held – clinical management and decision-making
- changes introduced by the new GP contract
- development plans to be addressed, perceived areas of unmet need
- new services, additional staff, constraints on change, use of practice performance indicators.

Thus, this approach involves a careful diagnostic phase. The implementation phase of the programme involved the setting up of a business group in each practice, representative of the main professional groups. Teams are encouraged to explore how they manage team meetings and a distinction is made between daily informal meeting opportunities, practice meetings where all groups are represented (perhaps monthly), whole practice meetings (perhaps twice a year), and small clinical case conference meetings involving some GPs and some professional staff. Conflict within the team is also addressed, particularly conflicts relating to identity, territory and control issues. This is one of the few team-building projects where conflict within teams is explicitly and carefully addressed. Practice management is also examined, particularly issues to do with leadership, performance monitoring, and decisions. Skills audits are also undertaken in order that resources available to teams can be clearly identified. Project work involves teams identifying particular issues which need addressing such as producing a weekly timetable of surgeries and room use, quarterly newsletter for staff, use of notice boards, links with social services and the role of a nurse practitioner. However, the approach tends to focus on specific single action issues and does not appear to provide explicit direction for developing primary health care strategy within local areas. The project also requires significant input from an external consultant for each team, with associated resource implications.

These examples of good practice describe the range of approaches taken to primary health care team building. They are by no means comprehensive, indeed the results of the review that was undertaken to substantiate this project revealed a wide variety of individuals and organisations offering team development approaches to primary care. Private consultants, clinical psychologists working within the National Health Service, occupational psychologists, departments of general practice, primary health care professionals, LOT members and professional associations were all involved in developing ways to promote teamworking within primary health care. What do these examples, as well as the responses of LOT members and our reviews of relevant literatures reveal? The final section of this report offers conclusions and a series of recommendations about team building in primary health care.

# Conclusions and recommendations

- *An enormous amount of work dedicated to building teamwork in primary health care has been conducted nationally in the United Kingdom. The work of local organising teams (LOTs) throughout the country has had a major impact in building more positive attitudes and perceptions among primary health care team members to their professional colleagues.* The value of this work cannot be overstated. It has washed across a large proportion of primary health care teams throughout the country, changing views of teamwork within them. LOT members have worked extremely hard, with limited resources and support, to increase co-ordination and collaboration in order to improve the quality of primary health care available to local people. Their approach has been professional and committed and, given the amount of support and the knowledge made available to them about team building, it is astonishing that so much progress has been made.

- *Various agencies, groups and individuals are involved in offering a wide variety of methods to those involved in the delivery of primary health care. However, they tend not to share a common conceptual frame of reference for teamwork and team building.* Their frames of reference are often drawn from practitioner literatures, rather than from evidence-based theory in organisational sciences. Many of the interventions used in team-building workshops lack empirical support for their effectiveness and their value is consequently unknown.

- *The first stage of awakening many primary health care teams to the concept of teamwork has been very successful, but there is now a need for new sophisticated approaches.* Many teams have made advances in sampling team-based working while addressing single issues such as health promotion, management of heart disease, management of diabetes. However, the major thrust should now be to encourage strategic teamwork. Primary health care teams must develop clear agreed strategies for addressing the health needs of local populations. This means they have to set aside time for planning, decision-making and reviewing their policies, practices and procedures, ideally adopting a continuous improvement orientation. Primary health care teams cannot meet the changing health care needs of local communities without a continual review of what those needs are, a continual review of their strategies for meeting those needs, and a continual review of the internal team processes (e.g. communication, decision-making, support for innovation) which underpin their efforts.

- *Many primary health care teams lack clear leadership and fail to take the time to hold even occasional regular team meetings to review their work.* How can they develop clear objectives or get feedback on their performance if, as organisations, they fail to set clear targets and objectives and to review their functioning on a regular basis? The history of organisational psychology has established an axiomatic principle that individuals, teams and organisations perform more effectively according to the extent that they define for themselves clear goals, targets and objectives.

- *An analysis of team needs prior to workshops requires pre-diagnostic work. Ideally instruments with high validity and reliability should be used to assess the needs of teams, or qualitative techniques which clearly indicate areas within which teamwork might produce more effective functioning.* In designing team-building workshops for primary health care teams it would be useful to consider four other important dimensions:

## 1. CLARITY OF TEAM OBJECTIVES

As indicated in the companion review (West and Slater, 1996), clarity of team objectives and feedback on team performance in relation to those objectives is of principal importance in influencing the effectiveness of primary health care teams. The design of team-building workshops should therefore incorporate some consideration of overall team objectives. There are two strategies: one is to focus on objectives in relation to specific actions, for example management of coronary heart disease; the other longer-term, and perhaps more promising strategy ultimately, is to encourage teams to develop objectives in terms of long-term strategies for dealing with health needs of populations. In other words, objectives can either be focused on single issues within teams, which may enable teams to avoid addressing broader issues of team functioning, or they can focus upon the overall objectives of the primary health care team and sub-objectives and tasks associated with those. Such an approach has been demonstrated to lead to significant improvements in team performance and productivity (Pritchard, 1991). The latter approach requires the primary health care team to address issues of leadership, management and decision-making within the team.

## 2. PARTICIPATION

A second issue to be addressed within teams is participation, which incorporates three sub-areas:

- interaction
- information sharing
- influence over decision-making.

In order for a team to function effectively the members must interact on a regular basis. Perhaps the most important way in which this is done is in formal *meetings with a clear agenda*. It is in such meetings that decision-making about the management of primary health care can effectively be made in the context of teamwork. Research on team functioning has shown that teams that take time out from their activities to review objectives, strategies and processes are more effective than those that do not (West, 1996). Where teams become so involved in the work and day-to-day demands that they are unable to take time out to review their work there is a danger of their focusing the allocation of their resources on non-priority issues.

*Information sharing and communication* are also important if members of the team are to effectively collaborate and co-ordinate their attempts towards promoting primary health care. Information and communication audits can be undertaken within teams to determine areas of deficiency and ways of overcoming them.

*Influence over decision-making* refers to the extent to which team members influence decisions about the strategies, objectives and processes of the team. A major problem in primary health care is that issues of leadership are obscured by anomalous structures. General practitioners are independent contractors and other members of the team are employees of a variety of organisations which differ depending on the profession of the team member. In one sense, the GP is the natural leader as the person to whom higher status is usually attributed. The lack of influence over decision-making felt by many primary care professionals in the areas of teamwork and the lack of clear team models in this domain, exacerbate difficulties caused by the historical separation of professional groups and leadership.

## 3. TASK ORIENTATION

An important component of team building is *task orientation* which is a team's ability to cope with conflicts of perspectives, views and opinions about appropriate objectives, strategies and processes. There is considerable evidence that constructive debate within teams aids effective functioning and promotes innovation. However, few team-building workshops address the management of constructive conflict effectively, though there are some notable exceptions in the LOT workshops. Team members should have the ability to identify constructive conflict, manage it effectively, identify destructive conflict and suppress it within their team's functioning. Where there are clear team objectives, and high levels of participation, task orientation provides an important safeguard against teams becoming so cohesive that agreements are seen as more important than good quality decision-making.

## 4. SUPPORT FOR INNOVATION

*Support for innovation* is the extent to which primary health care team members support the expression and application of ideas for new and improved ways of providing primary health care services. If primary health care is to develop, it is vital that new ways of doing things are trialled. Support for innovation exists when primary health care team members provide not only verbal support, but co-operate and give time and resources to the application of new ideas. Encouraging team members to develop a climate for innovation in primary health care is clearly important for the continued development of the services.

- *Primary health care team members require support and training to develop more sophisticated concepts of organisational functioning.* A problem encountered by those delivering team building to primary health care is the lack of knowledge that primary health care team members often have about teamwork in particular and organisational functioning in general. Issues commonly discussed within organisational settings such as objective setting, performance appraisal, feedback on performance and continuous improvement, are rarely addressed in the primary health care context.
- Perhaps the best opportunity for addressing this is the pre-qualification phase when inter-professional education could be undertaken to encourage members of different professions to begin working together in a training context to develop their knowledge of inter-professional collaboration and co-ordination. Post-qualification training would also be valuable in enabling primary health care team members to develop in their ability to work effectively as teams.
- *More radical approaches to team building might focus upon overcoming the organisational obstacles to effective teamwork in primary health care.* These include the status of GPs as independent contractors, the different lines of

33

management into primary health care teams, the lack of continuing support and education for teamwork in primary health care, and a lack of support for teams when primary health care team functioning is not adequate.

- *There is a need for those providing team building to consider carefully where to direct their energies.* Many teams have now experienced team-building workshops of a limited kind, focusing on specific issues. Those that have not may not be willing to participate at this stage. In the future, energy might perhaps best be focused on developing more effective teamwork by encouraging whole primary health care teams to commit time and energy to focusing on their overall objectives, strategies and processes in order that the effectiveness of primary health care can continue to be enhanced.

- *The overall aim should be to encourage a climate of reflexivity and continual improvement, building on the enormous motivation of primary care professionals to help those in their localities.* This is best achieved by coaching whole teams in the process of continually reflecting upon the team's objectives in meeting the health care needs of the population; team strategies for achieving their objectives; and team processes such as communication; decision-making and managing meetings. This reflection process should make clear where change is needed, which will enable professionals to use their resources most efficiently and effectively in promoting the health and wellbeing of those they help.

# Further reading

An excellent review of psychological research on teams in organisations is provided in the chapter by Guzzo and Shea (1992). *Groups That Work (and Those That Don't)*, edited by Hackman (1990), offers fascinating accounts of a variety of teams engaged in their daily work, such as cockpit teams, surgical teams and orchestras. *Effective Teamwork* (West, 1994) is a practical guide to effective teamwork, covering areas such as setting objectives, ensuring high levels of participation, encouraging team innovation and examining mental health in teams. Finally, *Group Processes: Dynamics Within and Between Groups* (Brown, 1988) is a readable and scholarly account of social psychological research on group functioning. For a comprehensive scientifically-oriented review of a wide range of issues related to work group psychology see *The Handbook of Work Group Psychology* edited by West (1996).

# References

Anderson, N. R. and West, M. A. (1994). *The Team Climate Inventory: Manual and Users' Guide*. Windsor, Berks: ASE Press.

Belbin, R. M. (1993). *Team Roles at Work: a Strategy for Human Resource Management*. Oxford: Butterworth Heinemann.

Boss, R. W. and McConkie, N. L. (1981). The destructive impact of a positive teambuilding intervention, *Group and Organizational Studies*, **6**, 45–56.

Brewer, N., Wilson, C. and Beck, K. (1994). Supervisory behavior and team performance amongst police patrol sergeants, *Journal of Occupational and Organizational Psychology*, **67**, 69–78.

Brown, R. J. (1988). *Group Processes: Dynamics Within and Between Groups*. London: Blackwell.

Cannon-Bowers, J. A., Salas, E., and Converse, S. A. (1993). Shared mental models in expert team decision making. In Castellan, N. J., Jr (ed.). *Current Issues in Individual and Group Decision-making*. Hillsdale, NJ: Lawrence Erlbaum, pp. 221–46.

Cordery, J. A. (1996). Autonomous work groups and quality circles. In West, M. A. (ed.). *Handbook of Work Group Psychology*. Chichester: Wiley.

Cotton, J. L., Vollrath, P. P., Froggett, K. L., Lengnick-Hall, M. C., and Jennings, K. R. (1988). Employee participation: diverse forms and different outcomes, *Academy of Management Review*, **13**, 8–22.

DeMeuse, K. P. and Liebowitz, S. J. (1981). An empirical analysis of teambuilding research, *Group and Organizational Studies*, **6**, 357–78.

Guzzo, R. A. (1996). Fundamental considerations about work groups. In West, M. A. (ed.). *The Handbook of Work Group Psychology*. Chichester: Wiley.

Guzzo, R. A. and Shea, G. P. (1992). Group performance and inter-group relations in organisations. In Dunnette, M. D. and Hough, L. M. (eds). *Handbook of Industrial and Organizational Psychology*, vol. 3. Palo Alto, Calif.: Consulting Psychologists Press, pp. 269–313.

Hackman, J. R. (1990) (ed.). *Groups That Work (and Those That Don't): Creating Conditions for Effective Teamwork*. San Francisco, Calif.: Jossey-Bass.

HEA (1995). *Multidisciplinary Team Workshop Programme: a Report on the Strategy and Development Workshop convened on 17 June 1994*. London: Health Education Authority.

Knapman, J., Morrison, T., Williamson, D., and Stamp, B. (1995). Teambuilding in primary care, *Primary Health Care*, **5**, 18–23.

Liebowitz, S. J. and DeMeuse, K. P. (1982). The application of team-building, *Human Relations*, **35**, 1–18.

Mullen, B. and Copper, C. (1994). The relation between group cohesiveness and performance: an integration, *Psychological Bulletin*, **115**, 210–27.

Nahavandi, A. and Aranda, E. (1994). Restructuring teams for the re-engineered organization, *Academy of Management Executive*, **8**, 58–68.

Pascale, R. T. (1990). *Managing on the Edge: Companies that Use Conflict to Stay Ahead*. New York: Simon & Schuster.

Pearson, C. A. L. (1987). Participative goal setting as a strategy for improving performance and job satisfaction: a longitudinal evaluation with railway track maintenance groups, *Human Relations*, **40**, 473–88.

Poulton, B. C. (1995). Effective Multidisciplinary Teamwork in Primary Health Care. PhD thesis. University of Sheffield.

Pritchard, R. D. (1991). *Measuring and Improving Organizational Productivity: a Practical Guide*. Praeger: New York.

Spratley, J. (1989). *Disease Prevention and Health Promotion in Primary Health Care: Team Workshops organised by the Health Education Authority*. London: Health Education Authority.

Stevens, M. J. and Campion, M. A. (1994). Staffing Teams: Development and Validation of the Teamwork – KSA test. Paper presented at the annual meeting of the Society of Industrial and Organizational Psychology, Nashville, Tenn.

Sundstrom, E., DeMeuse, K. P., and Futrell, D. (1990). Work-teams: applications and effectiveness, *American Psychologist*, **45**, 120–33.

Tannenbaum, S. I., Beard, R. L., and Salas, E. (1992). Teambuilding and its influence on team effectiveness: an examination of conceptual and clinical developments. In Kelly, K. (ed.). *Issues, Theory and Research in Industrial Organizational Psychology*. London: North Holland.

Tannenbaum, S. I., Salas, E. and Cannon-Bowers, J. A. (1996). Promoting team effectiveness. In West, M. A. (ed.) *Handbook of Work Group Psychology*. Chichester: Wiley, pp. 503–30.

Tziner, A. E. (1988). Effects of team composition on ranked team effectiveness. *Small Group Behavior*, **19**, 363–78.

West, M. A. (1994). *Effective Teamwork*. London: British Psychological Society.

West, M. A. (1996). Introducing work group psychology. In West, M. A. (ed.). *The Handbook of Work Group Psychology*. Chichester: Wiley.

West, M. A. and Poulton, B. C. (1995). Primary Health Care Teams: Rhetoric versus Reality. Paper not yet accepted for publication. Institute of Work Psychology, University of Sheffield.

West, M. A. and Slater, J. A. (1995). Teamwork: myths, realities and research, *Occupational Psychologist*, **24**, 24–9.

West, M. A. and Slater, J. A. (1996). *Teamworking in Primary Health Care: a Review of its Effectiveness*. Health Education Authority.

West, M. A., Poulton, B. C., and Hardy, G. A. (1994). *New Models of Primary Care: the Northern and Yorkshire Region Micropurchasing Project*. Harrogate: Northern and Yorkshire Region.

Woodman, R. W. and Sherwood, J. J. (1980). The role of team development in organizational effectiveness: a critical review, *Psychological Bulletin*, **88**, 166–86.

Yukl, G. and Vanfleet, D. (1992). Theory and research on leadership in organizations. In Dunnette, M. D. and Hough, L. M. (eds). *Handbook of Industrial and Organizational Psychology*, vol. 3. Palo Alto, Calif.: Consulting Psychologists Press, pp. 147–97.

# Appendix A
# How this review was conducted

## LITERATURE REVIEW

A literature review was carried out examining all books and journal articles published over a 15-year period from 1980 to 1995. The following databases were used:

- Medline – Index Medicus
- CINAHL – Cumulative Index of Nursing and Allied Health Literature
- ASSIA – Applied Social Science Index and Abstracts
- PsychLit – Psychological abstracts
- BIDS – Bath Information and Data Services – a national bibliographic database service for higher education
- NISS – National Information Services and Systems.

The initial search revealed little published work specifically referring to multidisciplinary teamworking or team building in primary care. Consequently researchers adopted a wider focus including combinations of the following key words: multidisciplinary, teamworking, health service, primary care, general practice, joint working, interdisciplinary, interprofessional, team building, team development, team effectiveness and interventions.

Relevant unpublished reports and in-house publications were also sought through contacts with appropriate individuals and organisations such as regional health authorities and university departments of general practice and primary health care.

## QUESTIONNAIRE SURVEY

Questionnaires were distributed to contacts in all known local organising teams (LOTs) in England, inviting views and opinions about multidisciplinary teamworking in primary health care. The survey was designed by the research team in collaboration with the HEA in order to gather information about teamworking and team building in primary health care in the UK. The participation of LOT members was voluntary and all answers were treated as confidential.

The questionnaire was divided into two sections. The first section concerned the effectiveness of teamwork in primary health care and LOT members' views of it. The second section was concerned with the approach that LOTs took to team building. Copies of the questionnaire were sent to all 70 local organising teams and 32 returned completed questionnaires. In addition consultancies involved in teamworking in primary care, departments of general practice in universities and many other relevant organisations (e.g. RCN, King's Fund, Health Visitors Association, Centre for the Advancement of Interprofessional Education) were invited to submit copies of publications, reports or programmes relevant to the enquiry into teamworking in primary health care.

The rather low response from LOTs appears to be due to the fact that not all LOTs are active at any given point in time. Attempts to prompt return of questionnaire by telephone calls to LOT representatives revealed that some had moved to other positions, were away on leave, or were no longer members of LOTs.

LOT representatives were asked to indicate the extent to which they thought multidisciplinary teamworking in primary health care could contribute to effectiveness in each of 19 areas (e.g. organisational efficiency, health promotion, patient care generally and role understanding across professional disciplines). They were also asked, in relation to the same 19 areas, to what extent they thought multidisciplinary teamworking had actually contributed to the effectiveness of primary care. LOT representatives were asked to identify what they saw as the main hindrances and enablers of effective teamworking in primary health care. They described any examples of outstanding teamworking in primary health care. Each respondent was also asked to estimate the percentage of primary health care teams in their area which were successful in building effective teamwork.

## INTERVIEWS

Interviews were conducted with 27 individuals, including representatives of local organising teams, consultants involved in promoting teamwork in primary health care, and members of departments of general practice. These interviews probed for further information about responses to the questionnaire and were directed to those who indicated their willingness to take part in such follow-up interviews.

# Appendix B
# The LOT Teamworking
# Questionnaire

**What is this survey?**
This questionnaire is a survey of your views and opinions about multidisciplinary team working in primary health care. It is not a test and so there are no right or wrong answers. The survey requires your personal views on the issues raised.

**Who is doing it?**
The survey has been designed by an independent research team from the University of Sheffield in collaboration with the HEA Multidisciplinary Team Workshop Programme, in order to understand more about team working and team building within primary health care in the UK.

**Do I have to fill this in?**
This survey is part of a research study designed to inform LOTs and those working within primary health care more generally about the extent and success of team working and team building. It is entirely voluntary.

**Who will see my answers?**
The completed questionnaires will be analysed at the University of Sheffield. All your answers will be treated as completely confidential and results will be grouped together so no individual's responses can be identified. This means that no one in the Health Education Authority or within your Local Organizing Team will be able to trace a response back to an individual.

**What feedback will I receive?**
Reports based on the survey as well as a broad literature review will be made available to all LOTs, as well as being more widely distributed.

**How do I fill in this survey?**
The questionnaire is divided into two sections. The first section concerns the effectiveness of team working in primary health care and your views of it. The second section is concerned with the approach that your LOT takes to team building. Some of the questions are of the form that require you to choose from amongst a number of alternatives and to tick appropriate boxes. Others are 'open ended' questions requiring you to provide a descriptive answer.

**How long will it take?**
The questionnaire will take about 45 minutes to complete. In general the first response that occurs to you is the best one to put down.

**What do I do if I don't know an answer?**
We would like you to answer every question. However if you really feel unable to give an answer, then please leave the question blank. If the question is not clear or you do not understand it, please telephone Michael West on 0114-275 6600.

**Now you have read the instructions, please begin the questionnaire.**

**Please tell us the name of your LOT** _____

*Team working in Primary Care*

**Section 1(a) – This section asks for your views about team working generally in Primary Care.**

1. To what extent do you think that multidisciplinary team working in primary care can contribute to effectiveness in the following area. Please circle the number which best represents your view.

| | | Very little contri-bution | Little contri-bution | Moderate contri-bution | Good contri-bution | Very great contri-bution |
|---|---|---|---|---|---|---|
| (a) | Growth and development of health professionals themselves | 1 | 2 | 3 | 4 | 5 |
| (b) | Organizational efficiency | 1 | 2 | 3 | 4 | 5 |
| (c) | Setting objectives | 1 | 2 | 3 | 4 | 5 |
| (d) | Decision making | 1 | 2 | 3 | 4 | 5 |
| (e) | Information sharing | 1 | 2 | 3 | 4 | 5 |
| (f) | Constructive debate | 1 | 2 | 3 | 4 | 5 |
| (g) | Support for new ideas | 1 | 2 | 3 | 4 | 5 |
| (h) | Monitoring of individual and team performance | 1 | 2 | 3 | 4 | 5 |
| (i) | Mutual respect across professional disciplines | 1 | 2 | 3 | 4 | 5 |
| (j) | Role understanding across professional disciplines | 1 | 2 | 3 | 4 | 5 |
| (k) | Health promotion | 1 | 2 | 3 | 4 | 5 |
| (l) | Disease prevention | 1 | 2 | 3 | 4 | 5 |
| (m) | Patient care generally | 1 | 2 | 3 | 4 | 5 |
| (n) | Needs assessment | 1 | 2 | 3 | 4 | 5 |
| (o) | Activity audit | 1 | 2 | 3 | 4 | 5 |
| (p) | Protocol development | 1 | 2 | 3 | 4 | 5 |
| (q) | Practice planning | 1 | 2 | 3 | 4 | 5 |
| (r) | Quality of care | 1 | 2 | 3 | 4 | 5 |
| (s) | Relationships with patients/ community | 1 | 2 | 3 | 4 | 5 |
| (t) | Appropriate skill use | 1 | 2 | 3 | 4 | 5 |
| (u) | Other areas (please specify) | 1 | 2 | 3 | 4 | 5 |

_____

_____

2. What do you see as the main hindrances to team working in primary health care?

   _____

   _____

3. What factors do you feel most enable effective team working in primary health care?

   _____

   _____

4. In your opinion, in what ways could effective teamwork improve and develop primary care?

   _____

   _____

5. Do you know of any examples of outstanding practice in terms of team working in primary health care?

   Yes ☐     No ☐

   If **YES**, please briefly describe

   _____

   _____

6. Would you be willing to describe in more detail these examples of outstanding practice in a follow up telephone interview with one of the researchers involved in this study? If so, please add your name and telephone number below.

   Yes ☐     No ☐

   Name  . . . . . . . . . . . . . . . . . . .   Telephone number  . . . . . . . . . . . . . . . . . . .

*Team working in Primary Care IN YOUR AREA*

**Section 1(b) – This section asks for your views about team working in Primary Care IN YOUR AREA.**

7. To what extent do you think that multidisciplinary team working in your area has contributed to the effectiveness of primary care on the following dimensions. Please circle the number which best represents your view.

|   |   | Very little contribution | Little contribution | Moderate contribution | Good contribution | Very great contribution |
|---|---|---|---|---|---|---|
| (a) | Growth and development of health professionals themselves | 1 | 2 | 3 | 4 | 5 |
| (b) | Organizational efficiency | 1 | 2 | 3 | 4 | 5 |
| (c) | Setting objectives | 1 | 2 | 3 | 4 | 5 |
| (d) | Decision making | 1 | 2 | 3 | 4 | 5 |
| (e) | Information sharing | 1 | 2 | 3 | 4 | 5 |
| (f) | Constructive debate | 1 | 2 | 3 | 4 | 5 |

| | | Very little contri- bution | Little contri- bution | Moderate contri- bution | Good contri- bution | Very great contri- bution |
|---|---|---|---|---|---|---|
| (g) | Support for new ideas | 1 | 2 | 3 | 4 | 5 |
| (h) | Monitoring of individual and team performance | 1 | 2 | 3 | 4 | 5 |
| (i) | Mutual respect across professional disciplines | 1 | 2 | 3 | 4 | 5 |
| (j) | Role understanding across professional disciplines | 1 | 2 | 3 | 4 | 5 |
| (k) | Health promotion | 1 | 2 | 3 | 4 | 5 |
| (l) | Disease prevention | 1 | 2 | 3 | 4 | 5 |
| (m) | Patient care generally | 1 | 2 | 3 | 4 | 5 |
| (n) | Needs assessment | 1 | 2 | 3 | 4 | 5 |
| (o) | Activity audit | 1 | 2 | 3 | 4 | 5 |
| (p) | Protocol development | 1 | 2 | 3 | 4 | 5 |
| (q) | Practice planning | 1 | 2 | 3 | 4 | 5 |
| (r) | Quality of care | 1 | 2 | 3 | 4 | 5 |
| (s) | Relationships with patients/ community | 1 | 2 | 3 | 4 | 5 |
| (t) | Appropriate skill use | 1 | 2 | 3 | 4 | 5 |

8.  What percentage of primary health care teams in your area would you say are successful in building effective team work?

    ☐ %

9.  In what ways have the primary health care teams in your area been most successful in improving team work?

    _____

    _____

    _____

10. In what areas of their work have the teams been least successful in making progress towards effective team work?

    _____

    _____

    _____

11. By what means does your LOT measure team working in primary health care? (Please include any documents, questionnaires, etc. which might illustrate your approach in your questionnaire return.)

    _____

    _____

    _____

12. By what means and on what dimensions does your LOT measure the effectiveness of primary health care generally?

   _____

   _____

   _____

13. Please add any other comments you may have, on issues to do with team working and effectiveness of primary health care below:

   _____

   _____

   _____

## Team Building

**Section 2 – The following section seeks information about the approach to team building you employ in your work with multidisciplinary teams in primary health care. The questions cover the methods used in your team building workshops, the content of the team building workshops, the attendees, the underlying principles and the effectiveness of the workshops.**

**What if you offer a range of different team building workshops/events?** If this is the case please respond to the following questions on the basis of your main, or most frequently used, type of workshop. *However, it is very important that we receive information from you about all the types of team building workshops/events that you run.* Please check that any documentation you send describing the other workshops/events also addresses the issues about content, attendance, effectiveness and evaluation raised in this section of the questionnaire. Thank you.

### Methods and Content

14. What are the overall aims of the team building workshops you run?

   _____

   _____

   _____

15. What are the main elements of the workshops?

   _____

   _____

   _____

16. To what extent do you cover the following areas in your team building workshops? Please indicate by circling the appropriate number.

|     |                         | Not at all | A little | Moderately | Quite substan-tially | Very substan-tially |
|-----|-------------------------|------------|----------|------------|----------------------|---------------------|
| (a) | Team objectives         | 1          | 2        | 3          | 4                    | 5                   |
| (b) | Health needs assessment | 1          | 2        | 3          | 4                    | 5                   |
| (c) | Health promotion        | 1          | 2        | 3          | 4                    | 5                   |

| | | Not at all | A little | Moderately | Quite substan- tially | Very substan- tially |
|---|---|---|---|---|---|---|
| (d) | Role clarification | 1 | 2 | 3 | 4 | 5 |
| (e) | Shared decision making | 1 | 2 | 3 | 4 | 5 |
| (f) | Innovations in practice | 1 | 2 | 3 | 4 | 5 |
| (g) | Team collaboration | 1 | 2 | 3 | 4 | 5 |
| (h) | Disease prevention | 1 | 2 | 3 | 4 | 5 |
| (i) | Relationships with patients | 1 | 2 | 3 | 4 | 5 |
| (j) | Relationships between professionals | 1 | 2 | 3 | 4 | 5 |
| (k) | Audit of activities | 1 | 2 | 3 | 4 | 5 |
| (l) | Protocol development | 1 | 2 | 3 | 4 | 5 |
| (m) | Practice planning | 1 | 2 | 3 | 4 | 5 |
| (n) | Computerisation | 1 | 2 | 3 | 4 | 5 |
| (o) | Getting to know one another as people | 1 | 2 | 3 | 4 | 5 |
| (p) | Building cohesion | 1 | 2 | 3 | 4 | 5 |
| (q) | Developing mutual role understanding | 1 | 2 | 3 | 4 | 5 |
| (r) | Team meetings | 1 | 2 | 3 | 4 | 5 |
| (s) | Communication | 1 | 2 | 3 | 4 | 5 |
| (t) | Commitment, i.e. time, resources | 1 | 2 | 3 | 4 | 5 |
| (u) | Others (please specify below) | 1 | 2 | 3 | 4 | 5 |

_____

_____

17. To what extent do you use the following in your team building workshops? Please indicate the percentage of workshop time taken up by:

(a)  Syndicate or small group exercises ☐ %

*Please describe the typical content areas*

_____

_____

(b)  Lectures ☐ %

*Please describe the typical content areas*

_____

_____

(c)   Other                                                            ☐ %

*Please describe the typical content areas*

_____

_____

## Attendance and Timing

18.  What percentage of primary health care teams in your area have taken part in the team building workshops?

☐ %

19.  How many people typically take part in a workshop?

☐

20.  Who typically attends the workshop sessions?

**Please tick as many boxes as apply**

(a)  The whole practice team (e.g. GP practice nurse, practice manager, receptionist)                         ☐

(b)  The whole practice team plus other community professionals (e.g. health visitors, district nurses, midwives)                ☐

(c)  The whole practice team plus a range of others (e.g. social workers, physiotherapists, chiropodists)                ☐

(d)  More than one whole practice team *how many teams typically* _____        ☐

(e)  Some members of the practice team                         ☐

(f)  Some members of the practice team plus other community professionals (e.g. health visitors, district nurses, midwives)    ☐

(g)  Some members of the practice team plus a range of others (e.g. social workers, physiotherapists, chiropodists)            ☐

(h)  Some members from more than one practice team *how many teams typically* _____        ☐

21.  If only some members of the practice team attend team building workshops, please tell us:

What disciplines typically attend?  _____

What percentage of the practice team typically attend?  ☐ %

22.  How long do the workshops usually last?  _____

23.  Is the team building programme

**Please tick**

Spread over a number of occasions?                         ☐

Completed in one session?                                   ☐

47

24. When do events typically take place? (Please tick)

    (a) ☐ Weekdays

    (b) ☐ Weekends

25. Where do the events typically take place? (Please tick as many boxes as apply)

    (a) ☐ Within the practices

    (b) ☐ In hotels

    (c) ☐ In other settings (Please specify) _____

26. Are there any follow-up events after the workshops?

    ☐ Yes    ☐ No

27. Who provides the input to the workshops? (Please tick as many boxes as apply)

    (a) ☐ LOT members

    (b) ☐ Outside lecturers

    (c) ☐ Others (If so, who) _____

**Effectiveness – This section concerns the effectiveness of the team building workshops you conduct.**

28. In your opinion, which elements of the team building workshops that you engage in are most effective and why?

    _____
    _____
    _____

29. Which elements of the team building workshops that you engage in are least effective and why?

    _____
    _____
    _____

30. In what ways do you think you could significantly improve the team building workshops you provide?

    _____
    _____
    _____

**Evaluation – This section concerns how you go about evaluating the team building workshop.**

31.   How do you evaluate the team building workshops? (e.g. participants' ratings, etc.)

_____

_____

_____

32.   On what dimensions are your team building workshops typically evaluated?

_____

_____

_____

33.   Do you have data available on participants' ratings?

☐ YES      ☐ NO

If YES, please send us copies if possible.

34.   Do you discern any consistent differences amongst professional groups in their evaluation of the workshops (e.g. GPs, health visitors)? If so, what are they?

_____

_____

_____

35.   Do you use standardized questionnaires, i.e. questionnaires which are widely used in multidisciplinary primary health care team settings such as the Team Climate Inventory?

☐ YES      ☐ NO

If YES, which instruments do you use?

_____

_____

_____

36.   When do you evaluate team building workshops?

(a)   ☐   After the workshop only

(b)   ☐   Before the workshop only

(c)   ☐   Both before and after the workshop

37.   If you conduct evaluations after, do you do these? (Please tick as many boxes as apply):

(a)   ☐   Immediately after

(b)   ☐   One week after

(c)   ☐   Three months after

(d)   ☐   Six months after

(e)   ☐   Other (please specify)

38. Overall to what extent do you feel that investment in team building provides results in terms of efficient and effective health services?

**Please Tick**

(a)  Very limited results  ☐

(b)  Moderate results  ☐

(c)  Quite good results  ☐

(d)  Very good results  ☐

(e)  Outstanding results  ☐

If you would like to make any further comments about this, please do so.

_____

_____

_____

_____

39. What do you think will be the key demands on primary health care teams in the future?

_____

_____

_____

_____

If you have any other comments you would like to make about team building in primary health care or the issues with which this questionnaire deals, please indicate these below.

_____

_____

_____

_____

Finally, if you have further comments you would like to make by telephone or in person; or if you wish to ask any questions about this survey, please telephone Professor Michael West on 0114 275 6600.

If you are willing to participate in a follow-up telephone interview please add your name and daytime telephone number below:

Name . . . . . . . . . . . . . . . . . . . . . .    Telephone number  . . . . . . . . . . . . . . . . . . . . . .
(include STD code)

**THANK YOU FOR YOUR CO-OPERATION**
**Please return the completed questionnaire and any relevant documents in the**
**pre-paid envelope provided.**